AROMATHERAPY & ESSENTIAL OILS FOR BEGINNERS

THE ULTIMATE GUIDE TO ESSENTIAL OILS FOR

HEALTH, BEAUTY & HOME

I0419394

Introduction

I want to thank you and congratulate you for downloading the book:

*"**Aromatherapy and Essential Oils for Beginners: The Ultimate Guide to Essential Oils for Health, Beauty and Home**"*. Aromatherapy has a long history dating back to the ancient Egyptians, who are believed to have created the first distillation device. It is also believed that they used oils infused with herbs in their rituals, perfumes, cosmetics and medicines.

Likewise the use of essential oils dates back at least a thousand years. In particular a French chemist named Rene Gattefosse discovered that lavender oil was a great healing tool when he, without thinking stuck his arm into a container of it after he sustained a bad burn. He was amazed when he noticed that the burn healed quickly and without scarring. He then began to study essential oils and is considered a pioneer in the field.

Since then, we have learned so much about the powerful benefits of essential oils and their ability to improve our health and wellness as well as home environment. I am excited to help you learn more about them and find new and useful ways to integrate them into your life. They provide wonderful natural remedies for so many of life's challenges.

I look forward to helping you begin this journey and wish you nothing but the best.

Chapter 1-

What exactly are Aromatherapy & Essential Oils?

Aromatherapy is simple at its core. It is the practice of using oils extracted from nuts, seeds, flowers, leaves, fruits, and twigs for special restorative purposes. These oils called essential oils, work in harmony with the body to produce powerful beneficial effects and have the ability to improve a person's well being both physically and mentally.

It has long been used to treat and relieve a variety of conditions including burns, infections, depression and high blood pressure among others. In addition, essential oils are known to have antibacterial properties when applied to the skin. One study discovered that when essential oils were inhaled, markers from the fragrance could be found in the blood, showing that aromatherapy was acting similar to a drug. Because of their special properties, the effects that the oils produce are difficult to replicate, and the benefits are most profoundly seen when using the essential oils.

The use of essential oils goes back thousands of years and is attributed to the Egyptians who used them for medicines, cosmetics and in their religious practices. Aromatic resins were also used in parts of the embalming process.

In addition to oils, aromatherapy uses other natural ingredients like vegetable oils, jojoba (a liquid wax), herbs, sea salts, clays and muds to achieve similar beneficial results. Aromatherapists may place the oils on the skin during a massage, or alternatively, use the oils as sprays or in diffusers to freshen their homes. There are various ways that the oils can be used:

> Indirect inhalation-person inhales the oils using a diffuser or by placing drops in a container in the room.
> Direct inhalation –person inhales the oils using an inhaler with drops floating on top of hot water. (ie: to treat a headache)
> Massage- essential oils are massaged into the skin.
> Mixing- essential oils are mixed into lotions, creams or bath salts.

The fragrance of the essential oil stimulates the nerves of the nose. The nerves send impulses to the brain that control memory and emotion. The effect of each oil is different, but generally, the oil will either be calming or stimulating.

There have also been many studies done to measure the effect of aromatherapy in cancer patients. The results show that aromatherapy may improve quality of life in patients with cancer. Some patients receiving aromatherapy have reported improvement in symptoms such as nausea or pain, and have lower blood pressure pulse, and respiratory rates. Studies of aromatherapy massage have had mixed results, with some studies reporting improvement in mood, anxiety, pain, and constipation and other studies reporting no effect. *

In 1998 a UK study looked at the effects of aromatherapy in 58 cancer patients. Most of these patients were women with breast cancer who said that they would like aromatherapy to help them with feelings of stress, anxiety, depression and fear. Each patient had 6 aromatherapy treatments during the study. At the end of these treatments all the patients showed a significant improvement in their feelings of anxiety, depression and stress.**

*cancer.org

**cancerresearchuk.org

Chapter 2

Starting to use essential oils

Getting treatment from an aromatherapist

When they are being massaged into the skin, essential oils are usually blended with another oil called a carrier oil. It is usually a vegetable oil and is called a carrier oil because of its ability to carry oil to the skin. Essential oils are especially concentrated and if used directly on the skin could cause damage. This is why the carrier oil is needed.

The most common types of carrier oils are:

Olive oil

Jojoba oil

Almond oil

Grapeseed oil

Avocado oil

Coconut oil

When you have your first aromatherapy massage, the aromatherapist will probably ask you about lifestyle and health. If you have a serious or complicated medical condition, they may ask to speak with your primary doctor to make sure it's medically advisable for you to receive aromatherapy treatment. The aromatherapist will choose the oils that they know will help your specific condition and help manage your symptoms the best. They will massage the oils gently into your skin. The session will normally last between an hour and a hour and a half. They may play relaxing music during the session as well. It is usually a very calming and relaxing experience.

Using essential oils at home

When you are at home and want to make your own aromatherapy treatment, it is relatively easy to do so. You can add essential oils to water and use an oil burner to inhale them. Adding the essential oils to hot or boiling water is a great method for getting started. This is a great way to relieve a sinus headache, or a blocked or stuffy nose. You can also add a few drops to a cloth or handkerchief and inhale them this way.

You can also add a few drops to your bathwater. This method has been effective at easing anxiety, insomnia or general stress relief. However, it is wise to consult with an aromatherapist before adding essential oils to your bath due to risk of skin irritation.

There are also a multitude of other ways to use essential oils to improve your health, home and environment. The great benefit of essential oils is that they allow you a natural way to clean and deodorize your home and help heal your body at the same time! There are very few other things that are as versatile.

Here are a few ways to use essential oils at home:

Plug in air freshener-If you have a glass plug in air freshener that's empty, essential oils are a great way to create a natural refill. Remove the wick with a large knife. Fill up the reservoir half way with a favorite essential oil. Next add some filtered water to fill it up to the top. Replace the wick and then plug it in normally. Refilling your plug in this way is not just a money saving strategy, but it's a healthier option to the ingredients in the original air freshener.

Homemade fabric freshener-If you like to use Febreze or any of the other fabric fresheners then the good news is you can make your own fabric fresheners using essential oils. The benefit is that you have control over the ingredients being used, and you are saving money as well. To get started you will need:

> Empty spray bottle (16 oz. or larger)
> 1 tbsp. baking soda
> 2 cups filtered water
> 10 drops of essential oil

Mix the baking soda and essential oil on a small plate. You may need a fork to mix thoroughly. Add the mixture to the spray bottle and then pour in the water. Gently shake the mixture before you use it. You can choose one scent or mix for a unique blend.

Natural carpet deodorizer-Add 5-6 drops of your favorite essential oil to 1 cup of baking soda. Mix the baking soda and oil together, then add to a shaker. Think of a parmesan shaker (a parmesan shaker or similar may work well). Sprinkle on your carpets and then let it sit for 15-20 minutes. Vacuum as usual. The baking soda will absorb all the bad odors, and the oil will deodorize. Voila!

Killing Mold-Don't you hate the mold that you see living in the cracks and crevices of your tub and shower? I know I do. The good news is there is an easy solution. Tea tree oil is a great essential oil to use to kill this yucky mold and have a clean shower in no time. Simply mix 1 tsp. of tea tree oil and 1 cup of water in a spray bottle. Spray the affected area and then let it dry. Don't wipe it off. You should see an improvement shortly.

Mice repellant-Mice hate the smell of peppermint. This is a good thing that you can use to your advantage. Simply mix 2 teaspoons of peppermint oil with one cup of water in a spray bottle. Spray the mixture anywhere you have seen mouse activity or where you believe mice have been. The best part is you don't have to deal with strong toxic chemicals used in commercial mouse traps.

Antibacterial room spray-By creating your own room spray you are not only able to get the scent you love, but you are saving money as well. To do this, simply mix 10 drops of your favorite essential oil with 1 cup of filtered water in an empty spray bottle. Spray it anytime you feel the room needs refreshing. You can also spray this on the toilet to get a great antibacterial benefits of this.

Bathroom deodorizer- Simply spray one or two drops of essential oil into the toilet paper roll before putting it in the holder. Then every time you move the roll, you will get fresh burst of the new scent.

Sleep aid-If you have trouble sleeping or even if you don't, this is a great tip to try. Lavender is a great sleep inducing scent that is a natural way to help with any sleep problems you may have. Mix 10 drops of lavender oil with filtered water and put it into a spray bottle on the fine mist setting. Then spray your bedsheets and pillow cases 30 minutes before you go to bed. This is enough time so that your sheets aren't damp, but will still allow the scent to be fresh enough to lull you to peaceful sleep.

Furniture spray- Instead of buy commercial spray, you can make your own. It's easy to do with essential oils. Simply mix 2 teaspoons olive oil, ½ teaspoon lemon oil, ¼ cup vinegar, and

1 3/4 cups filtered water into a spray bottle. Shake it up to mix all ingredients and spray on furniture as needed.

Keeping fruit fresh- To keep your fruit from spoiling so quickly, fill a bowl with cool water and 2-6 drops of Lemon. Drop washed fruit into the water and stir. Your fruit will be luscious for days longer than usual.

Rid the house of pet odors- Geranium and Lemongrass essential oils are great for dispersing unwanted pet odours. A traditional burner masks the aroma quite well, but sometimes to really tackle the problem you need to get down to their level – on the floor.

Add about 10 drops of your preferred essential oil to a half-filled bucket of hot water and your regular cleanser, and mop around the areas where pet odors are the most intense.

*Allergies-*If you're like me and you have allergies, then you understand how terrible it can be. One natural remedy for treating allergic nasal reactions is to rub some lavender oil on your palms (you could also use a handkerchief or tissue) and inhale deeply.

*Underwear drawers-*To keep drawers fresh, (pun intended), place a drop of your favorite essential oil onto a cotton ball or piece of tissue and put it in the drawer. Whenever you open the drawer the scent will be fresh and delightful. For a sensual smell try Ylang ylang, Sandalwood, Jasmine or Rose. For a more conservative scent, try Lavender or Geranium.

Disinfect your sponge- Add Lemon oil to your kitchen sponge between use to disinfect it.

Relief of cramps- If you are woman who suffers from cramps every time Aunt Flo comes to town, you'll be happy to know that you can find natural relief with essential oils. First mix one part Clary Sage, Basil or Rosemary oil with four parts carrier oil. Massage into your abdomen and cover with a warm cloth compress. Repeat as needed.

Disinfect cuts- Mix either Lavender oil or Tea tree oil with a carrier oil in equal parts and apply to the affected area.

Chapter 3

Blending Essential Oils

Blending essential oils

Different oils can be blended together to create what is called a synergy. This means that the powers of the oils change to enhance their energy and potency. When a level of potency has been reached, you achieve synergy. Recipes for blending must be followed exactly, and then the mixture should be left to age for at least 1 week before adding them to carrier oils for use.

There are several things to remember when you are blending essential oils. Here are some questions to ask yourself:

1. What result are you looking for?
2. What notes does each oil have?
3. Will each oil blend well with the other?

Let's get started answering these questions and understanding blends a bit more.

Essential oils can be categorized together based on their aromas. There are several different categories:

- *Floral*
  (i.e. Lavender, Neroli, Jasmine)

- *Woodsy*
  (i.e. Pine, Cedar)

- *Earthy*
  (i.e. Oakmoss, Vetiver, Patchouli)

- *Herbaceous*
  (i.e. Marjoram, Rosemary, Basil)

- *Minty*
  (i.e. Peppermint, Spearmint)

- *Medicinal/Camphorous*
  (i.e. Eucalyptus, Cajuput, Tea Tree)

- *Spicy*
  (i.e. Nutmeg, Clove, Cinnamon)

- *Oriental*
  (i.e. Ginger, Patchouli)

- *Citrus*
  (i.e. Orange, Lemon, Lime)

Oils that are in the same category generally blend well together. This is a general rule, and you can successfully blend oils from different categories together. But in general, here are some rules.

- Florals blend well with spicy, citrusy and woodsy oils.

- Woodsy oils generally blend well with all categories.

- Spicy and oriental oils blend well with florals, oriental and citrus oils. Be careful not to overpower the blend with the spicy or oriental oils.

- Minty oils blend well with citrus, woodsy, herbaceous and earthy oils.

Have you ever noticed that a fragrance smells differently when you first spray it than it does hours later? This is because some oils evaporate more quickly than others, and as the oils evaporate, this changes the fragrance of the remaining oils in the blend.

 There are different classifications of oils, based on how quickly they evaporate. The oils that evaporate the fastest are called top notes. These usually evaporate in 1-2 hours. They also usually have antiviral properties and are light, fresh and invigorating in nature. They give the first impression of the blend and are generally less expensive. The oils that evaporate between 2-4 hours are called middle notes. They normally give body to the blend and have a balancing effect. They are normally warm and soft in nature. Oils that evaporate the slowest are called base notes. They are very heavy and very solid in nature. They are normally intense and heady and they slow down the evaporation of the other oils. They are the most expensive of all the oils. Some base notes can take several days to fully evaporate. Below you will find a chart of oils and their corresponding classifications:

Top Notes	Middle Notes	Base Notes
Basil (Top to Middle)	Bay	Balsam Peru
Bergamot (Top to Middle)	Black Pepper	Cassia (Base to Middle)
Cajuput	Cardamom	Cedarwood
Cinnamon	Chamomile	Cinnamon (Base to Middle)
Clary Sage (Top to Middle)	Cypress	Clove
Coriander (Top to Middle)	Fennel (Middle to Top)	Frankincense

Eucalyptus	Geranium	Ginger (Base to Middle)
Grapefruit	Ho Leaf	Jasmine
Hyssop (Top to Middle)	Ho Wood	Myrrh
Lemon	Hyssop (Middle to Top)	Neroli (Base to Middle)
Lemongrass (Top to Middle)	Juniper	Oakmoss
Lime	Lavender (Middle to Top)	Patchouli
Mandarin / Tangerine	Marjoram	Rose
Neroli (Top to Middle)	Melissa (Middle to Top)	Rosewood (Base to Middle)
Verbena	Myrtle	Sandalwood
Niaouli	Nutmeg	Valerian

Orange	Palma Rosa	Vanilla
Peppermint	Pine	Vetiver
Petitgrain	Rosemary	Ylang Ylang (Base to Middle)
Ravensara	Spikenard	
Sage	Yarrow	
Spearmint		
Tagetes		
Tangerine		
Tea Tree (Top to Middle)		
Thyme (Top to Middle)		

*deancoleman.org

Blending tips

**

When creating a new blend, start out small with a total number of drops of either 5, 10, 20 or 25 drops. 25 drops should be the most that you start with. By starting small, you waste less oil in your blending experiments.

Start creating your blend by only using essential oils, absolutes or CO2s. After you have designed the blend, then you can dilute it by adding carrier oils, alcohol, etc. If you hate the blend you created, you have then not wasted any carrier oils or alcohol.

Keep a journal that lists each oil that you used with the number of drops used for each creation. When the creative juices flow, it is easy to get carried away and later forget the exact recipe for your blend; one drop too much or too little of even one oil can drastically change the aroma of your blend. When you find that perfect blend that you love, you want to be able to reduplicate it, and it's near impossible if you didn't take notes! If you are especially ambitious, it's also a wise idea to note the vendor name of the oil that you used as the aroma and quality of oils do vary between vendors (even with the same vendor, the aroma of oils can vary from batch to batch, due to crop fluctuations and resourcing).

To store your beautiful creations, perfume sample bottles and 2ml amber "shortie" bottles are very inexpensive and can often be purchased from aromatherapy vendors and glass bottle companies.

Be sure to label your blends clearly. If you don't have enough room to specify exactly what your blend is, label it with a number that corresponds to a number in your notebook.

Start off your experiments by creating blends that are made up in the following ratio (you do not have to be exact – this is just a guideline to get you started): 30% of the oils are top notes, 50% are middle notes, and 20% are base notes. See the chart above to find out what oils belong to each category.

Some oils are much stronger than others, especially the absolutes and CO2s. Study oils you wish to use in a given blend and observe the oils that have the strongest aromas. Unless you want those oils to dominate the blend, you will want to use dramatically less of the stronger oils in your blend.

To learn more about the strength of oils, it is useful to experiment. Begin by adding one drop of a selected essential oil to 4 drops carrier oil. This will result in a 20% dilution. Smell it and study the aroma. To obtain a 10% dilution, add 5 more drops of carrier oil. Smell it, study the aroma again, then repeat as desired. This can help educate you on the characteristics and strengths of each essential oil at various dilution ratios.

After creating your blend, allow it to sit for a few days before deciding if you love or hate it. The constituents (natural chemicals) contained within the oils will get cozy with each other and the aroma can change, usually filling out more over time.

**aromaweb.com

Chapter 4

Essential oil recipes

Base Perfume Recipe

7-15 drops of your perfume blend

1 tablespoon Jojoba (other carrier oils may be substituted, but stable carrier oils with longer shelf lives are recommended)

Directions: Blend all oils together well and store in an airtight dark-colored glass container. Dab a drop onto your pulse points. Please note that this blend has a heavy concentration of essential oils and is meant to be used sparingly. As with any new oils and blends that you use, you must check all safety data for the oils in your blend and do a skin patch test prior to using.

Alcohol/Water Base Perfume Recipe

4 1/4 teaspoons Vodka

1 1/2 teaspoons Distilled Water

30 drops of your perfume blend

Directions: Blend all ingredients well and store in an airtight 1 ounce dark-colored glass container. Let sit for two weeks, shaking the bottle 1-3 times daily (more often is better) to mix the oils. After two weeks has passed, filter the perfume through a coffee filter and rebottle (using the same bottle is fine). Please note that this recipe has a heavy concentration of essential oils and is meant to be used sparingly. As with any blends that you use, you must check all safety data for the oils in your blend and do a skin patch test prior to using.

Cologne Recipe

4 1/2 teaspoons Vodka

2 teaspoons Distilled Water

22 drops of your perfume blend

Directions: Blend all ingredients well and store in an airtight 1 ounce dark-colored glass container. Let sit for two weeks, shaking the bottle 1-3 times daily (more often is better) to mix the oils. After two weeks has passed, filter the cologne through a coffee filter and rebottle into a one-ounce, fine-mist sprayer bottle. Please note that although this recipe makes a lighter cologne, it still has a heavy concentration of essential oils and is meant to be used sparingly. As with any blends that you use, you must check all safety data for the oils in your blend and do a skin patch test prior to using. This makes only a one-ounce quantity so that you can try your cologne to see if you like it or want any changes to it before making a larger quantity.

Body Splash Recipe

4 1/2 teaspoons Vodka

2 teaspoons Distilled Water

14 drops of your perfume blend

Directions: Blend all ingredients well and store in an airtight 1 ounce dark-colored glass container. Let sit for two weeks, shaking the bottle 1-3 times daily (more often is better) to mix the oils. After two weeks has passed, filter the body splash through a coffee filter and rebottle into a one-ounce, fine-mist sprayer bottle.. As with any blends that you use, you must check all safety data for the oils in your blend and do a skin patch test prior to using. This makes only a one-ounce quantity so that you can "try" your body splash to see if you like it or want any changes to it before making a larger quantity.

Essential oils dilution

You must remember that essential oils are powerful. You should treat them the same way you treat a medicine. This is not meant to scare you away from using oils, because they can bring wonderful benefits to you life and wellness. But you should respect the oils and recognize that they should not be treated lightly. You should almost always dilute any essential oil you are using and not put it directly on your skin undiluted.

There is a risk of sensitization if you use oils undiluted. Sensitization is similar to an allergic reaction that can result in itchy skin or a rash like reaction. More severe cases of sensitization can lead to respiratory problems or anaphylactic shock.

In general, a 2% dilution is considered safe practice for adults and with oils that don't have a more stringent dilution protocol. For children and elderly people, cut the dilution in half. For children, use only essential oils designated as safe for children unless you are very well versed in aromatherapy protocols for children.

A good rule of thumb is when making 2% dilution blends, is to measure the oil by the drop. Generally speaking, adding 12 drops of oil to each fluid ounce (30 ml) of cold pressed carrier oil, lotion, vegetable butter or other natural moisturizer will give you the proper ratio.

Once you have chosen your essential oil, you can dilute it by adding it to various base products such as unscented bath gels, hand and body lotions, and massage lotions to name a few. Below you will find some general rules of thumb for creating custom essential oil dilutions.

Massage.......................... 5 drops per tsp. of base oil or lotion

Inhalation....................... 1-2 drops in boiling water or on a tissue

Light Bulb Ring............... 1-2 drops

Bath............................... 8-10 drops in bath water

Sauna............................. 2 drops to 2 ½ cups water

Facial............................. 2-3 drops in base product

Foot Bath....................... 8 drops in bowl of water

Facial Sauna................... 10 drops in bowl of water

Cleanser......................... 20 drops in 4 ounces of base product

Body............................... 5-15 drops in base product

Chest Rub....................... 10-20 drops to 1 oz of carrier oil

Washing Machine.......... 10-20 drops per load

Auto Vent Outlet........... 2-3 drops

By now you should be getting a feel for how essential oils work and hopefully are getting excited about using them in various ways and creating your own special custom blends. I also wanted to share with you some recipes that can help you improve your health and wellbeing.

Recipes for Anxiety:

Blend #1

2 drops Bergamot

2 drops Clary Sage

1 drop Frankincense

Blend #2

3 drops Sandalwood

2 drops Bergamot

Blend #3

3 drops Lavender

2 drops Clary Sage

Blend #4

1 drop Rose

1 drop Lavender

2 drops Mandarin

1 drop Vetiver

Essential Oils for Weight Loss:

Peppermint

Peppermint oil has a refreshing scent. Just dilute a few drops before a meal to reduce hunger and appetite.

You can also add a couple of drops to water for added energy and appetite suppressant.

You can also add a few drops to suppress cravings and have an energizing start to your day.

Lemon

Daily massaging of lemon oil helps to eliminate toxins that are stored in the skin and waste stored in fat cells.

Adding 1 or 2 drops of essential oil to your water before breakfast will gently detoxify the body. You can also inhale or diffuse lemon oil before meals.

Bergamot

Place a few drops in a cloth and inhale to relieve stress when you are tempted to continue eating.

You can place a drop in one tsp. of honey or drink a 4oz. of coconut milk for a calming effect.

It can be diluted in a warm bath to assist with stress and start a refreshing day.

Recipes for headaches

If you are prone to get headaches or migraines try some of these essential oil recipes for fast natural relief. Try rubbing this natural headache home remedy into your temples and the back of your neck to soothe tension and ease pain.

Natural headache balm

1/4 cup Shea Butter

1 tablespoon Beeswax, grated

1 tablespoon Grapeseed oil OR
Herb infused oil (see below)

1/4 teaspoon (or 1 capsule) Vitamin
E

One of the Essential Oil blends
below

Soothing Lavender Blend

8 drops Lavender essential oil
1 drop Jasmine essential oil
1 drop Chamomile OR Lemon Balm
essential oil

Reviving Peppermint Blend

6 drops Peppermint essential oil
2 drops Rosemary essential oil
1 drop Eucalyptus essential oil

Place the shea butter, beeswax and grapeseed oil in the top part of a double boiler, warming slowly over a low heat until they're melted.

Remove from heat and add the essential oils and vitamin E.

Pour into a dark glass or plastic jar. Store in a cool, dark place.

Headache Buster Blend*

30 drops Peppermint

30 drops Lavender

10 drops Frankincense

10 drops Wintergreen

10 drops Birch

Put into a 1/3 oz. glass roller and top off with fractionated coconut oil. Rub into temples, forehead and back of neck. Reapply as needed.

*RichestoRagsbyDori.blogspot.com

Chapter 5

Essential Oils Glossary*-

Allspice Berry - This oil has a warm, spicy-sweet aroma. It is used in spicy or masculine scents. It combines well with orange, ginger, patchouli and all of the spice oils including cinnamon, cassia and clove. Aromatherapy benefits: warming, cheering, comforting, nurturing.

Anise - The oil of anise and star anise are often used and sold interchangeably because they are similar in aroma and chemical make-up. The primary constituent of both is anethole, a sweet substance that solidifies at room temperature. If this happens simply warm the bottle in a warm water bath until the oil liquefies. Aromatherapy benefits: cheering, mildly euphoric.

Basil, Sweet – There are many types of basil: linalool basil, exotic basil and sweet basil. The odor of the linalool type is very green, floral-sweet and is most often used in expensive perfumes. The exotic type of basil is stronger with a hint of camphor. Frontier's sweet basil type combines both qualities in a floral-spicy aroma with a lasting herbal sweetness. Clary sage, bergamot and lime oil work well with basil oil. Aromatherapy benefits: clarifying, uplifting, energizing, refreshing.

Bay Laurel Oil- is sometimes known as *Laurel Leaf Oil*. Is great for encouraging confidence, fortitude, inspiration, protection, direction and creativity.

Bergamot-The aroma of Bergamot Essential Oil is reminiscent to that of orange, but it is more complex and almost has an underlying floral characteristic to it. It may be helpful in use during periods of depression and is known for its ability to help combat oily skin and acne.

Citronella- It is known for being citrusy, slightly fruity, fresh, sweet. It is commonly used for excessive perspiration, fatigue, headache, insect repellant, and oily skin.

Cardamom Seed - The oil has a spicy, camphor-like aroma with floral undertones. It imparts a warm note to masculine scents and floral perfumes. It blends well with bergamot, frankincense, ylang ylang, cedarwood and coriander. Aromatherapy benefits: warming, comforting, alluring.

Cedarwood, Red - Red cedarwood essential oil actually comes from a type of juniper known as Juniperus virginiana, whose common name is eastern red cedar. The balsamic-woody aroma of cedarwood oil evokes a feeling of inner strength and centeredness. It is quite useful in times of emotional stress and anxiety to overcome feelings of powerlessness.

Chamomile, Roman - Roman chamomile contains only trace amounts of the intense blue component azulene, which gives German chamomile its color. This oil is commonly used in perfumery. It blends well with bergamot, jasmine, neroli and clary sage, lending a warm, fresh note when added in small quantities. The aroma is not long-lasting like that of the German chamomile but it is a mild, soothing oil. Aromatherapy benefits: relaxing, calming.

Cinnamon Bark - Also known as Ceylon cinnamon, this is the true cinnamon of world commerce. Its aroma is similar to cassia, or Chinese cinnamon. The aroma of Ceylon cinnamon is preferred to cassia for perfume where it gives a warm, floral-enhancing effect. Cinnamon oil blends well with oriental-woody notes and is often combined with frankincense. It is a skin irritant and should be handled with care. Aromatherapy benefits: comforting, warming.

Clary Sage - Clary sage oil has a spicy, hay-like, bittersweet aroma. It combines well with coriander, cardamom, citrus oils, sandalwood, cedarwood, geranium and lavandin. The aroma of clary sage is long-lasting and the oil is valued as a fixative for other scents. Aromatherapy benefits: centering, euphoric, visualizing.

Fennel, Sweet - Sweet fennel oil has a very sweet, earthy, anise-like aroma due to its primary constituent, anethole. Sweet fennel usually contains more anethole than bitter fennel oil. Aromatherapy benefits: nurturing, supportive, restorative.

Frankincense - Various species of frankincense trees grow wild throughout Western India, Northeastern Africa and Southern Saudi Arabia. The oil is distilled from the gum resin that oozes from incisions made in the bark of the trees. The oil is spicy, balsamic, green-lemon-like and peppery. It modifies the sweetness of citrus oils such as orange and bergamot. It is also the base for incense type perfumes and is important in Oriental, floral, spice and masculine scents. Aromatherapy benefits: calming, visualizing, meditative.

Geranium (Bourbon) - This oil is one of the most important perfumery oils and is an important ingredient in all types of fragrances. It has a powerful, leafy-rose aroma with fruity, mint undertones. Bourbon oil, from the island of Reunion, is considered the finest grade, and has the best staying power. It is used in skin care products for both its fragrance and its toning, cleansing properties. Aromatherapy benefits: soothing, mood-lifting, balancing.

Hyssop - Historically, hyssop herb was regarded as a sacred plant and was used as a strewing herb and incense to purify holy places. The scent of the oil is reminiscent of the herb; spicy, sweet, woody and strong. It blends well with clove, lavender, rosemary, myrtle, sage, clary sage and citrus oils. Aromatherapy benefits: refreshing, purifying.

Lavender - Lavender oil is used in baths, room sprays, toilet waters, perfumes, colognes, massage oils, sachets, salves, skin lotions and oils. It has a sweet, balsamic, floral aroma which combines well with many oils including citrus, clove, patchouli, rosemary, clary sage and pine. Aromatherapy benefits: balancing, soothing, normalizing, calming, relaxing, healing.

Lemon – Lemon oil that is cold pressed, is much better oil than distilled. The scent is evocative of the fresh ripe peel. Lemon oil in the bath or in massage oils should be well diluted as it can cause skin irritation. Caution: avoid using the oil in body care products when going out into the sun as it can cause redness and burning of the skin. Aromatherapy benefits: uplifting, refreshing, cheering.

Lemon Eucalyptus - The aroma of Eucalyptus citriodora is similar to the aroma of citronella. Both contain citronellal as a major component. Eucalyptus citriodora has a fresh, rosy, grass-like aroma. It blends well with eucalyptus globulus, moderating that oils somewhat medicinal aroma. Aromatherapy benefits: purifying, invigorating.

Lime - Two types of lime oil are commonly sold: distilled and cold-pressed. Distilled oil is pale yellow or clear in color with a perfumey-fruity, limeade aroma. Pressed oil, which we offer, is yellowish to green in color, with a rich, fresh, lime peel aroma. While pressed lime oil is produced in smaller quantities and is more expensive than distilled lime oil, it is preferred in aromatherapy. Lime oil applied to the skin, may, in the presence of sunlight, cause a skin reaction. Aromatherapy benefits: refreshing, cheering.

Marjoram, Wild - Wild marjoram oil is not a variety of marjoram but is actually distilled from a species of wild thyme which grows in Spain. The oil has a strong, sweet-spicy, eucalyptus fragrance and is used in small amounts in massage oils for its invigorating effect. Aromatherapy benefits: purifying, clarifying.

Myrrh - Natural myrrh resin is one of the oldest known perfumery materials. The oil has a balsamic, warm and spicy aroma that blends well in Oriental, woody and forest-type perfumes. It is also used in ointments and other skin care products. Myrrh was used as incense and in embalming preparation in ancient Egypt. Aromatherapy benefits: centering, visualizing, meditative.

Neroli - Oil of neroli is distilled from the flowers of the bitter orange tree. It has a very strong, refreshing, spicy, floral aroma and is one of the most widely used flower oils in perfumery. It is an ingredient in eau de cologne and blends well with citrus oils and floral oils. Neroli is also used in premium natural cosmetic preparations such as massage oils, skin creams and bath oils. Aromatherapy benefits: calming, soothing, sensual.

Orange, Mandarin - Although the botanical differences between mandarin and tangerine are slight, the oils expressed from each differ in aroma and are not considered interchangeable in aromatherapy. The floral, neroli-like undertones of mandarin are evocative and sensual. Mandarin is used in combination with other citrus oils in colognes and fantasy-type perfumes. Aromatherapy benefits: uplifting, cheering, sensual.

Oregano - Oregano has a strong, herbaceous, green-camphoraceous, medicinal top note. The middle note is spicy, medicinal. The dry out is sweet-phenolic woody, bitter-sweet. Oregano essential oil is invigorating, purifying and uplifting.

Patchouli - Used in countless perfumes and fragrances, patchouli is noted for its long-lasting fragrance and fixative ability. It borders on the exotic and even the name patchouli evokes images of heady aromas, dark, rich colors, candlelight, incense and intrigue. The aroma is very intense; it can be described as earthy, rich, sweet, balsamic, woody and spicy. Patchouli oil is one of the few essential oils that improve with age. Aromatherapy benefits: romantic, soothing, sensual.

Peppermint - Peppermint has a powerful, sweet, menthol aroma which, when inhaled undiluted, can make the eyes water and the sinuses tingle. Aromatherapy benefits: vitalizing, refreshing, cooling.

Pine - Pine oil is distilled from the twigs and needles of the Scotch pine that grows throughout much of Europe and Asia. It has a fresh, resinous, pine needle aroma. The oil is used to scent a number of household and personal care products such as room sprays, detergents, vaporizer liquids, cough and cold preparations and masculine perfumes. When used in skin care preparations, pine oil should always be well diluted as it can be irritating to sensitive skin. Aromatherapy benefits: refreshing, invigorating.

Rose Otto - Rose oil is one of the oldest and best known of all the essential oils. The fragrance of rose is associated with love. It is warm, intense, immensely rich and rosy. It is used in perfumes to lend beauty and depth. A drop or two in a massage, facial or bath oil is luxurious and soothing. The oil is used in skin creams, powders and lotions. Aromatherapy benefits: romantic, supportive, gently uplifting.

Rosemary - Rosemary is known as the herb of remembrance. The plant produces an almost colorless essential oil with a strong, fresh, camphor aroma. It's used in many citrus colognes, forest and Oriental perfumes, and eau de cologne. Rinses for dark hair often contain rosemary, as do room deodorants, household sprays, disinfectants and soaps. Aromatherapy benefits: clarifying, invigorating.

Rosewood - Rosewood, or bois de rose, is a tropical tree growing wild in the Amazon basin. It has a sweet-woody, floral-nutmeg aroma that finds extensive use in fantasy-type perfumes and colognes. It is also used to scent soaps, creams, lotions, bath oils and massage oils. Aromatherapy benefits: gently strengthening, calming.

Sandalwood - Sandalwood oil has a sweet-woody, warm, balsamic aroma that improves with age. The essential oil blends wonderfully with most oils, especially rose, lavender, neroli and bergamot. Sandalwood oil is also an excellent cleansing, astringent addition to massage and facial oils, bath oils, aftershaves, lotions and creams. Aromatherapy benefits: relaxing, centering, sensual.

Tangerine - It is an orange-colored oil with the vibrant fragrance of fresh tangerines. The oil is used in colognes and occasionally in perfumes.(See Mandarin Orange.) Aromatherapy benefits: cheering, uplifting.

Tea Tree - The leaf of the tea, or ti, tree had a long history of use by the indigenous peoples of Australia before tea tree was "discovered" by the crew of the famous English explorer James Cook. The aroma of the oil is warm, spicy, medicinal and volatile. It is occasionally used to scent spicy colognes and aftershaves. It blends well with lavandin, rosemary and nutmeg oils. Aromatherapy benefits: cleansing, purifying, uplifting.

Thyme, Red - Red thyme oil is the natural essential oil produced from wild-growing thyme plants. It has an intense, sweet, herbal, spicy-medicinal aroma. Both red and white thyme are used to scent soaps, colognes and aftershaves. Caution: Thyme oil can be irritating to the skin and should be used cautiously. Aromatherapy benefits: cleansing, purifying, energizing.

Thyme, White - White thyme starts out as red thyme oil that has been further refined and redistilled to remove the constituents that produce the red color. The aroma and action of white thyme oil are a bit milder than that of red thyme. Both are used to scent soaps, colognes and aftershaves. Caution: Thyme oil can be irritating to the skin and should be used cautiously. Aromatherapy benefits: cleansing, purifying, energizing.

Vanilla - The aroma is lingering sweet balsamic. Aromatherapy benefits: calming, comforting, balancing.

Vetiver - The aroma is rich, woody, earthy and sweet. It improves with age. Vetiver oil is used extensively in perfumery for its fixative effects as well as its fragrance. Aromatherapy benefits: supportive, grounding.

Ylang Ylang Extra - Ylang ylang oil is distilled from the early morning, fresh-picked flowers of the cananga tree. The distillation process is interrupted at various points and the oil accumulates is removed. The first oil to be drawn off is the highest quality and is graded "extra." Ylang ylang extra has an intense floral, sweet, jasmine-like, almost narcotic aroma. Aromatherapy benefits: sensual, euphoric.

*Auracacia.com

Partial list of medical conditions and what oils to avoid:

If you are pregnant: avoid Basil, Cedarwood, Clary, Coriander, Hyssop, Jasmine, Juniper, Marjoram. Oregano, Myrrh, Peppermint (which should also be avoided while nursing), Rockrose, Rosemary, Sage, and Thyme.

If you are pregnant, it is generally safe for you to use the following oils in moderation.

Oils that are safe for you to use while pregnant:

As long as your pregnancy is going well, it's fine for you to use:

citrus oils, such as tangerine and neroli

German camomile

common lavender

frankincense

black pepper

peppermint

ylang ylang

eucalyptus

bergamot

cypress

tea tree oil (not in labour)

geranium

spearmint

If you suffer from a seizure disorder: it's best to avoid Basil, Fennel, Hyssop, Rosemary, and Sage.

If you have high blood pressure: Pine, Rosemary, Sage, and Thyme.

Best places to purchase essential oils online:

> Edensgarden.com
> Auracacia.com
> Planttherapy.com
> Edenbotanicals.com

Conclusion

Thank you again for downloading this book! I hope you have found a new appreciation for Essential oils and some great home health remedies that you can incorporate into your life. I hope that this is just the beginning of your use of Essential oils and Aromatherapy, and I wish you nothing but health and happiness.

All the best,

Isla

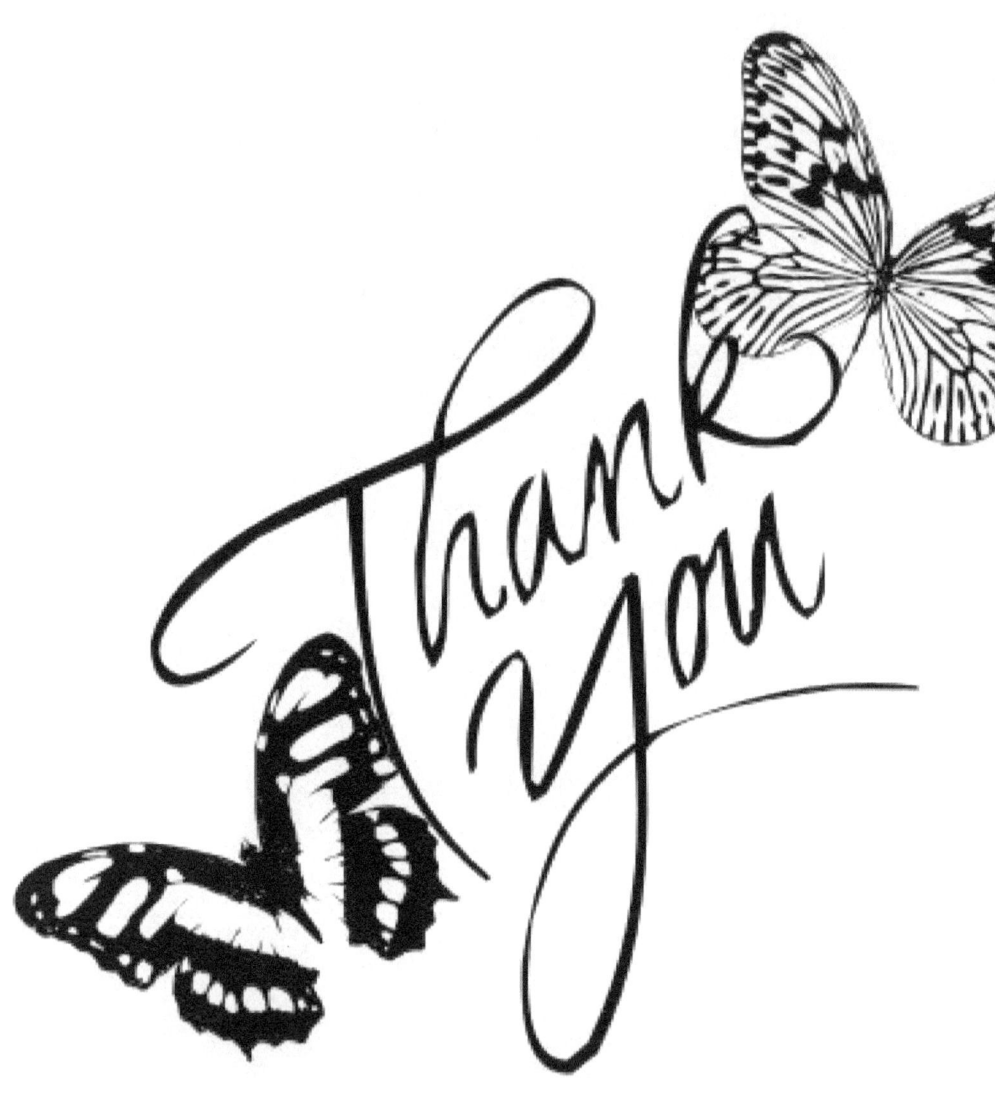

Finally, if you enjoyed this book, then I'd like to ask you for a favor, would you be kind enough to leave a review for this book on Amazon? It'd be greatly appreciated!

Thank you and good luck!

Preview of 'Essential Oils for Weight Loss: Easy Ways to Supercharge your Weight Loss Success with Essential Oils'

Essential Oils to Boost Weight Loss

In your weight loss journey, you will find several essential oils that will provide you with that added boost to push you towards reaching your goals. There are several essential oils that are excellent for boosting weight loss efforts. The beauty of essential oils is that they each have different properties and can produce different results. You can also try blending different oils together to harness and combine the different properties of the oils to achieve a variety of benefits.

Additionally, essential oils can be combined with aromatherapy in order to boost your weight loss. Aromatherapy stimulates parts of the brain that have positive effects on our emotional, physical and mental state. Breathing in fragrances stimulates the amygdala and the hippocampus which are the centers of human emotions and memory. Inhaling essential oils also stimulates brain receptors responsible for blood pressure, heart rate, attention span, stress and motivation.

Essential oils can provide an excellent supplemental boost to your weight loss plan. Many times, the struggle to lose weight has more to do with our psychological hurdles and burdens than it does with physical issues. Essential oils are great in this way because they can help you overcome some of the emotional or psychological blocks that have prevented successful weight loss in the past. For example, whether the issue is cravings for sweets, emotional eating, dieting fatigue, lack of motivation or slow metabolism, there is undoubtedly an essential oil or combination of oils that will alleviate the issue. Essential oils could be the missing ingredient that you need to finally achieve your weight loss goals.

Below you will find a list of essential oils and their properties and best uses for weight loss:

Grapefruit oil

Grapefruit oil is possibly the best essential oil to use to increase weight loss results. It suppresses appetite, boosts energy, reduces the appearance of cellulite, prevents bloating and dissolves fat. It contains nootkatone which is a natural chemical compound that stimulates a particular enzyme (AMPK specifically) which controls the body's energy levels and metabolism. AMPK hastens chemical reactions in the brain, liver and skeletal muscles. Research has shown that AMPK and nootkatone interact that results in improved endurance, reduced weight gain, decrease in body fat and increased physical performance.

It is also believed that limonene, a key hydrocarbon component found in grapefruit, creates lipolysis, a process where body fat is broken down and dissolved.

How to use it

Internally

Drink one glass of water with 1 or 2 drops of grapefruit essential oil. Be sure to buy high quality oil that is specifically made for internal use. It will help to get rid of toxins, lose excess fat, and weight management. You should aim to drink it in the morning so that you will benefit from its effects throughout the day.

Note: When ingesting essential oils, it's best to mix 1 or 2 drops with 1 tsp. of honey then add to warm water. This ensures safe absorption and processing by your body.

Massage

Add a few drops to a carrier oil such as extra virgin olive oil or unrefined virgin coconut oil. Massage it into into areas where fat accumulates thoroughly (about 30 minutes) and leave it on for a few hours before rinsing off.

Bath

Add 5 drops of grapefruit essential oil to you bath. Combine it with:

5 drops of ginger

5 drops of orange

5 drops of lemon

5 drops of sandalwood

Add a cup of apple cider vinegar

This combination will not only smell wonderful, but provides an excellent cellulite bath to aid with reducing the appearance of cellulite. Soak for approximately 30 minutes.

Caution: Always do a patch skin test first before applying any oil to the skin. You want to be sure that you are not allergic to any oil or oil combination before using them topically.

Lemon oil

This oil can be used to suppress appetite, increase energy and improve digestion. It aids the body in getting rid of toxins that would otherwise be stored in the fat cells. It has lots of great benefits aside from weight loss. When used as a mood enhancer, it is excellent at alleviating negative feelings. It also increases levels of norepinephrine a stress hormone which controls our fight or flight responses. In addition, norepinephrine increases oxygen in the brain for better brain function and improves blood flow and heart rate for optimal muscle functioning. In addition, lemon oil used in conjunction with grapefruit oil increases lipolysis.

Lemon oil is also good for getting rid of intestinal parasites, which contribute to weight gain.

How to use it:

Internally

Add 1 or 2 drops of lemon oil honey then to water in the morning before breakfast. This will help your body jumpstart your digestion and eliminate excess toxins.

Daily Massage

Add a few drops to a carrier oil of your choosing and massage into fat prone areas once per day. Helps eliminate toxins.

Please visit the kindle store for the rest of this book.

Check out my other books

Simply Bliss: Easy Ways to Organize and De-Stress Your Life Forever

Meditation for Beginners: How to Meditate to Decrease Stress and Vastly Improve Health & Happiness

Positive Affirmations: Positive Affirmations for Health and Wealth that Will Transform Your Life Forever

www.ingramcontent.com/pod-product-compliance
Lightning Source LLC
Chambersburg PA
CBHW030542290526
45786CB00004B/1817